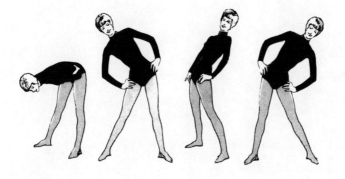

Illustrations by Diego Caillet

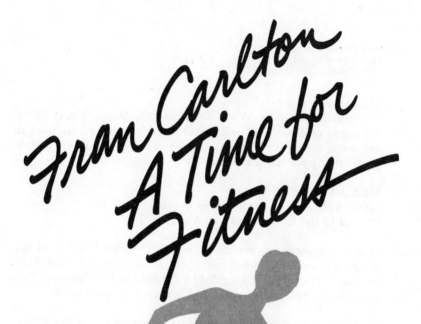

Fran Carlton
A Time for Fitness

A DAILY EXERCISE GUIDE FOR THE CHRISTIAN

WORD BOOKS, PUBLISHER
WACO, TEXAS

First Printing, July 1976
Second Printing, August 1976
Third Printing, December 1977

ISBN 0-87680-464-4
Library of Congress catalog card number: 76–5719
Printed in the United States of America

Scripture quotations are from the King James Version of the
Bible unless otherwise marked. Quotations marked *Living Bible*
are taken from *The Living Bible, Paraphrased* (Wheaton: Tyn-
dale House Publishers, 1971) and are used by permission.

Grateful acknowledgment is made to the publisher for permission
to reprint from "Stopping by Woods on a Snowy Evening" from
The Poetry of Robert Frost edited by Edward Connery Lathem.
Copyright 1923, © 1969 by Holt, Rinehart and Winston. Copy-
right 1951 by Robert Frost. Reprinted by permission of Holt,
Rinehart and Winston, Publishers.

To
Lynne and Julie

Contents

Part One

YOU ARE A MAGNIFICENT CREATION

The photographs in
Part I are by the author.

I.

In His Own Image

You are magnificent! You are created in the image
of one who is perfect. No matter how many lunar
modules, no matter how many space capsules, no
matter how many complicated computers man may
devise—he can never equal God's creation of
the human body.

You! You are truly magnificent! God gave you
that magnificent body and then he gave you the
ability *and* the responsibility to take it and make
of it whatever you will. God's gift to you is your
body, your life. Your gift to him is what you make of
that life, that body.

In Genesis we are told of God's creation: "And God
said, Let us make man in our image, after our likeness:
and let them have dominion over the fish of the sea,
and over the fowl of the air, and over the cattle, and
over all the earth, and over every creeping thing that
creepeth upon the earth. So God created man in his
own image, in the image of God created he him; male
and female created he them" (Gen. 1:26–27).

Do you remember studying the structure of the human eye in your high school biology class? You probably spent several weeks on the intricacies of the eye and you still didn't understand it all! Just one small part of the body and yet so complex, so magnificently designed, so awe-inspiring!

Did you ever stop to consider that inside you there are approximately sixty *thousand* miles of blood vessels busily carrying life-sustaining blood to every part of your body? The average adult body has approximately ten pints of blood; that incredible little pump that is no bigger than a large fist and weighs less than a pound—your heart—pushes that ten pints of blood through more than one thousand complete circuits every day, a total volume of five to six thousand quarts of blood.

The master plan for you is something phenomenal. You house over 600 muscles and 206 bones—unless you are that one of every twenty people who has an extra bone—an extra rib. (This happens three times more often in men than in women. I wonder—could there be any connection between this physiological phenomenon and the rib that God took from Adam to make Eve?)

The most amazing thing of all about you is that in all the world you are unique! There are over 3 billion people on this earth, and yet in all these masses—indeed throughout history—there has never been, nor will there ever be, another you. God doesn't have a mass production assembly line. You are one of a kind. You are special! The psalmist describes it beautifully: "You made all the delicate, inner parts of my body, and knit them together in my mother's womb. Thank you for making me so wonderfully complex! It is amazing to think about. Your workmanship is marvelous—and how well I know it!" (Ps. 139:13–14, *Living Bible*).

As I am writing I can look out and see the marvelous Atlantic Ocean. It is especially beautiful today. There is some wind and the surf is "up," as the surfers would say. There is something about the roar of the ocean that is far more relaxing than any tranquilizer could ever be for me. I come here often, and yet I never cease to be totally in awe of God's handiwork. I find myself singing:

O Lord my God, when I in awesome wonder
Consider all the worlds thy hands have made,
I see the stars, I hear the rolling thunder,
Thy power throughout the universe displayed,
Then sings my soul, my Savior God to thee;
How great thou art, how great thou art!*

I am so deeply humbled before Him and wonder why He cares for me, or for that matter, for any of us! Yet He has given us *dominion* over the works of His hands:

"When I consider thy heavens, the work of thy fingers,

---

*From "How Great Thou Art," © Copyright 1953 by Stuart K. Hine, Assigned to Manna Music, Inc. © Copyright 1955 by Manna Music, Inc., 2111 Kenmere Ave., Burbank, CA 91504. International Copyright Secured. All Rights Reserved. Used by Permission.

the moon and the stars, which thou hast ordained; What is man, that thou art mindful of him? and the son of man that thou visitest him? For thou hast made him a little lower than the angels, and hast crowned him with glory and honor. Thou madest him to have dominion over the works of thy hands; thou hast put all things under his feet" (Ps. 8:3–6).

We also find a description of man's creation in Genesis 2:7: "And the Lord God formed man of the dust of the ground, and breathed into his nostrils the breath of life; and man became a living soul."

When God made man, maybe He should have put a maintenance manual in the glove compartment! Our bodies were designed in such a way that they *require* a certain amount of physical activity in order to keep functioning properly. We are made of sturdy stuff, with the capability of doing hard physical labor all day, *every* day.

Not too many years ago our way of life required a great deal of physical activity from us, but not any more. We have become an inactive, spectator-oriented society. We are over-weight and under-exercised! We ride when we could walk. We watch when we could participate. We complain because we are so tired, and yet we have done nothing exhaustive. Nothing physically exhausting, that is. But we *really* are tired!

If you owned a very valuable piece of machinery that required regular lubrication and maintenance in order to keep it running properly and that machine was

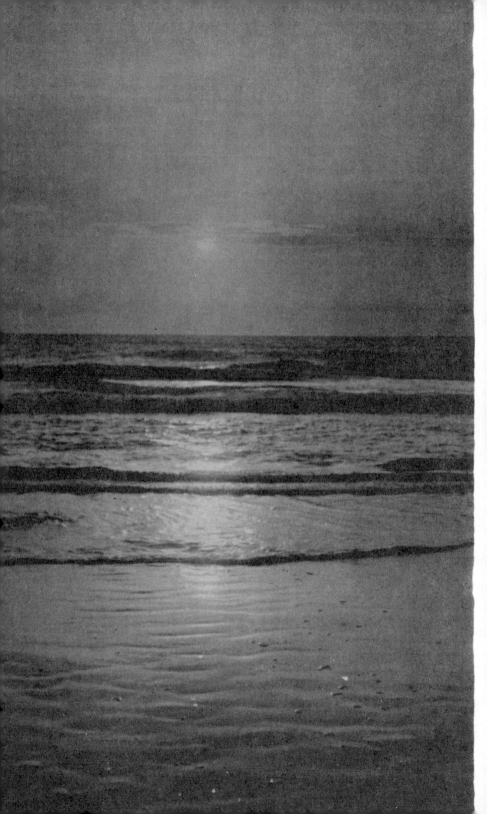

irreplaceable and important to your business, you would see to it that the lubrication and maintenance were done, wouldn't you? It would be utterly foolish to allow something so very important to you to go to rust and ruin.

Your body and your health are the most important things you have. *Knowing* that regular exercise is necessary for the maintenance of that magnificent machine, does it still make sense if you neglect it?

Did you brush your teeth today? Why did you brush them? Well, there are many good reasons, but probably the real reason is that it has become a habit.

I have two teen-age daughters. I don't have to remind them to brush their teeth any more, but oh, how well I remember the days when I did. Every morning as they were leaving for school, the scene went something like this: "Julie, did you brush your teeth?" Up until Julie was about eleven or twelve years old the answer was most often, "No, Mom, I forgot." So, "Go back and do it!" I *saw* to it that Lynne and Julie developed that habit of brushing their teeth! I would guess that the scene has been, or is, much the same at your house.

All of us have been "conditioned" to brush our teeth. Getting the exercise that you need each day must become just as much a part of your day, just as much a daily habit, as brushing your teeth. Actually, that exercise program is far more important to you. Now, I am not suggesting that you stop brushing your teeth: by all means keep right on doing that. Just understand the necessity of regular exercise as a daily health habit.

You are tired, you are tense, because you have *not* done anything physically taxing. The normal, natural way to release tensions from the body is through physical activity. Through exercise! The way to unwind, to relax, to be able to *rest,* is to get the exercise you need.

Exercise is essential for keeping the vital organs in condition. The heart is a muscle that improves with conditioning, indeed *requires* exercise, to keep it functioning properly.

The heart and the bloodstream are perhaps the most vital of our vital systems. Consider the work they perform: The circulatory system carries oxygen to *every* cell of the body and brings back waste materials to be disposed of. Processed energy is also carried to all parts of the body by the circulatory system. If we consume more energy than we need our body stores it for future use.

Unfortunately for the sake of our appearance and our health, the body knows only one way of storing excess energy—in the form of FAT (I do believe that is the ugliest word in the English language) to be taken out of storage when needed and used to keep the engine running. Most of us never give the system a chance to draw on that reserve supply. We just keep on adding more. The result is an overweight, unattractive body and an overworked heart and circulatory system. For every extra pound of fat in storage, your body adds seven to nine *miles* of blood vessels that the heart must pump blood to.

The bloodstream also carries and distributes the

hormones that determine so many functions of the body, and those all-important white corpuscles that help keep us healthy by fighting infectious diseases.

This magnificent machine *must* have regular maintenance!!

Exercise is essential for good digestion and good elimination. Exercise is essential for maintaining muscle tone and endurance. Without exercise muscles become weak and flabby, and joints get out of balance. Exercise is essential for promoting restful sleep. (If you *wake up* tired, it is probably because you went to bed tense; you did not release those tensions through exercise. There is a great deal of difference in being physically tired and in being emotionally and mentally tired.) Exercise is essential for the normal release of tension. If you want to look, to feel, and to function as you were designed to—as God intended you to—you must make a habit of regular exercise!

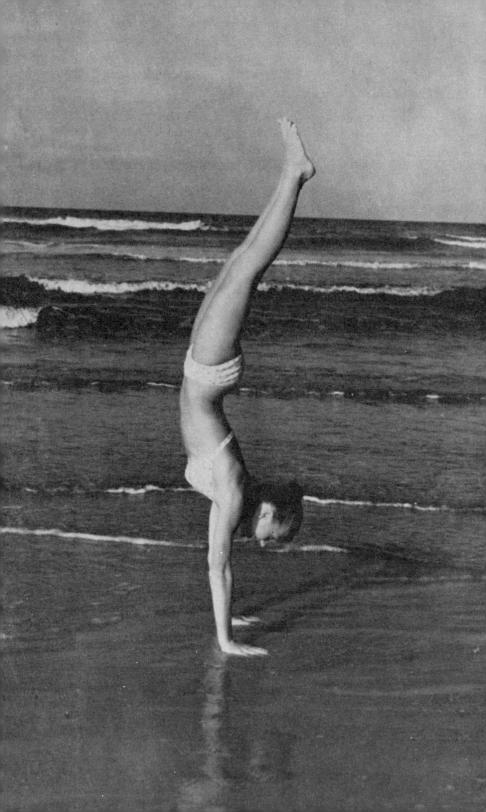

II.

His Temple

"What? know ye not that your body is the temple of the Holy Ghost which is in you, which ye have of God, and ye are not your own? For ye are bought with a price: *therefore glorify God in your body,* and in your spirit, which are God's" (1 Cor. 6:19–20, italics mine). Is there any way that it could be made clearer than that?

"Know ye not that ye are the temple of God, and that the Spirit of God dwelleth in you? If any man defile the temple of God, him shall God destroy, for the temple of God is holy, which temple ye are" (1 Cor. 3:16–17). ". . . For ye are the temple of the living God" (2 Cor. 6:16).

Take a good long, honest look at your body. Does it *glorify* God? Is it a *fit* place for him to dwell?

An old farmer once said: "It ain't what you know so much as what you *do* that counts." I know from my own experience what it is like to be overweight. The writer of Deuteronomy could have been describing me when he said, "Thou art waxen

fat, thou art grown thick, thou art covered with fatness"
(32:15). When I was expecting our first child, I was inactive for the first time in my life. Like so many women,
I used my "condition" as an excuse to eat more. I have a
weakness for chocolate candy and for books, so I ate
candy bars and read all day. Now, I had a degree in
physical education; I knew more exercises than anybody
needs to know. I had had courses in nutrition. I *knew*
what I should be doing. But what I was doing—was
reading and eating chocolate candy! Paul described
it so well in Romans 7:19: "For the good that I would,
I do not; but the evil which I would not, that I do."

What happened to me is the same thing that happens
to most overweights. Gaining weight is a gradual process,
and, somehow, before you fully realize what is hap-
pening, it has already happened! *After* Lynne was
born, I weighed 170 pounds (today I weigh 116 to 118).
It seems that many women who are overweight start
with their first pregnancy, gaining too much weight and
never quite getting rid of it. Soon after Lynne was
born, a friend took a picture of me and that beautiful child. When I saw the picture, I was just like
the prodigal son—I "came to my senses" (Luke 15:17,
Living Bible). Somehow, in the picture I could see
what I had been telling myself just wasn't there in
the mirror. I began practicing what I *knew* I should
have been doing all along—that is, exercising regularly
and eating sensibly.

It took me several months of proper diet and exercise
to get down to my normal weight. But I had learned

my lesson! Today, I believe that God allowed me to have that experience so that I could better understand and help others. I only regret that I burned that picture and don't have the evidence to share with you.

By the way, I *still* have a weight problem. I gain weight very easily and must stay on a very-low-calorie diet to maintain my desired weight. This has become a way of life for me. In Colossians 3:10 (*Living Bible*) Paul says: "You are living a brand new kind of life. . . ."

When you accept the challenge to "glorify God in your body," you will indeed be living a brand new kind of life! I eat the foods that I know my body needs and don't eat the "stuff" I don't need— *and* I exercise every day to maintain the machine. I try to *do* what I *know*.

If you are overweight, I plead with you to *do* what *you* know. Romans 14:20 (*Living Bible*) says: "Don't undo the work of God for a chunk of meat." (Nor, I might add, for a slice of Key lime pie, either.) With Christ as your strength you cannot fail.

"Whether therefore ye eat, or drink, or whatsoever ye do, do all to the glory of God" (1 Cor. 10:31) .

III.

Promises to Keep

The woods are lovely, dark and deep,
But I have promises to keep,
And miles to go before I sleep.

These lines from Robert Frost's poem "Stopping by
Woods on a Snowy Evening" are a special favorite
of mine.

We all have "promises to keep." Promises to keep
to our families, to our friends, to those people we
love—we owe it to them to be the very best that
we can be. Why is it that we make such an effort to
look our best, to be kind, thoughtful, and considerate
when we are among strangers, people who really
are not that important to us; and then when we are
at home with the people who mean so much to us
we are at our worst? Don't the people you love
have a right to expect from you the very best that you
can be? If you are not the best person that you can
be, you are cheating them.

You have promises to keep to yourself! Your

self-image is so important to you. Many volumes have been written on the subject. "You are what you think you are," we are told over and over. Proverbs 23:7 says: "For as he thinketh in his heart, so is he." If you *know* what you should be doing and you are *not* doing it—you are cheating yourself. That is the very last person you want to cheat! Shakespeare said it beautifully: "This above all else to thine own self be true." You may lie to the world and get away with it. But you cannot successfully lie to yourself. You owe the very best that you can be to yourself!

You have promises to keep to your Creator, to Him who made you in His own image. God has a right to expect from you the very best that you can be. If you are not doing what you *know* you should be doing— you are cheating God!

William N. Thomas said: "Perhaps the only good and perfect gift that we can give to the world is ourselves at our best." If you are not striving to be the very best that you can be, you are cheating those people that you care about, you are cheating yourself, and you are cheating your God. "Yes, each of us will give an account of himself to God" (Rom. 14:12, *Living Bible*).

You have promises to keep.

IV.

The Very Best That You Can Be

Close your eyes for a moment and visualize yourself at
your very best. At your optimum weight, with no
bulges, with curves where curves ought to be,
muscles toned and firm, posture tall and regal. You
move easily, gracefully, and confidently. "And God
saw every thing that he had made, and, behold,
it was very good" (Gen. 1:31). In his book *Being Me*,
humorist Grady Nutt repeatedly says: "I'm me, I'm
good, 'cause God don't make *no junk.*" Indeed he
does not!

The physical potential of the human body is beyond
our comprehension. It wasn't so very long ago that
the entire world watched the Olympics on television, when, for all the world to see, a tiny Russian
girl performed physical feats that were previously
considered impossible. I knew that it was impossible as
did scores of others; but somebody neglected to tell
Olga that it couldn't be done. She *believed* she could—
and she *did!* What is more, she performed with such
grace, such form, such apparent ease that it was

breathtakingly beautiful to behold. That day, Olga expanded the realm of physical potential just a bit.

In light of the physical potential of the human body, it really doesn't seem like much to expect that we would at least "maintain the machine." We cannot all be Olympic stars. We can be aware, however, of the extraordinary physical potential that was given to each of us, and we can at *least* get the physical activity, the daily exercise that our bodies must have if we are to experience life at its best—if we are to *look* our best, *feel* our best, *be* our best.

It is not too late to begin. Through my fitness clinics, classes, and television programs, I have seen many neglected, tired, prematurely aging bodies become revitalized and resculptured, self-images improved, and a sense of well-being regained.

Here are a few comments from a number of women who have found that they can, indeed, look better, feel better, and like themselves better by making a time for fitness a daily habit.

Dear Fran,
I sure do enjoy your exercise program. I have gained unbelievable results in such a short time. . . .

Dear Fran,
I have been intending to write you ever since I took the course you offered in Clearwater. It made such a change in my looks and my feelings that I have preached your daily exercises wherever I go.
A very good friend of mine whom I don't see

very often wanted to know what I had done to look
fifteen years younger. You can bet she is now doing
your exercise program.

We vacationed in New Orleans this summer (I
lived and worked there years ago and this was my
first trip back). All my friends were amazed at how
young and trim I looked. They had all gotten fat.
Did I ever feel good! . . .

Dear Fran,
My friend and I have been using your exercise
record and it has done wonders for us.
Thank you . . .

Dear Fran,
I am 66 years old, and after 45 years of smoking,
I gave them up last Thanksgiving, which was fine
but I put on 10 pounds in 2 months, which scared
me because I can't afford to go on those diets,
and so one day, bless you, you came on the air and
made it sound so simple, and at home alone I wasn't
embarrassed if I did look like a fool. So I tried and as
you say I couldn't lift a foot off the floor—my feet
were like lead. My waistline creaked like it needed
oiling. *But*, now after 3 months I can do all those
exercises, not with your grace, but I manage. I
have lost the 10 pounds, taken off 3 inches from
my waist, and I even have an ankle now. As you
always say, I feel better and look better, and even
like myself better. So, thank you, Fran, from an old
but very grateful fan of yours. . . .

Dear Fran,
I will always sing your praises loud and clear
for I know and appreciate the help you offer. I hope

that more people will discover your wonderful program and how much good your exercises will do for them. . . .

Dear Fran,
   I follow your program all the time and enjoy it so much. I feel so much better since I've taken the time to exercise daily. . . .

Dear Fran,
   I want to thank you for what you have done for my figure. I really think your exercises are superb. . . .

Dear Fran,
   I would like to wish you and your family a very Merry Christmas. Thanks to you I am having a much happier one. I have been exercising for over a year now. I have also watched the calories and lost weight. After my son was born I weighed 156 pounds. Before, I weighed 135 pounds at 21 years of age. So you can understand how I felt. Also I was a physical disaster. Now I am as fit as I was in High School and I only weigh 125 pounds. Now—120 would be a perfect weight for me. I hope to attain that weight soon with your help.
   Thanks for changing my life. . . .

A healthy, attractive body can be yours. It will require daily dedication. You must make your fitness time a daily habit; as much a part of your routine as brushing your teeth. Set a specific time each day when you will exercise. If this means getting up a half hour earlier or using part of your lunch hour to exercise, I can assure you that it will be more than worth the effort. Only you can make that visualization of yourself at your very best become a reality!

"And so, dear [ones], I plead with you to give your bodies to God. Let them be a living sacrifice, holy— the kind he can accept. When you think of what he has done for you, is this too much to ask?" (Rom. 12:1, *Living Bible*).

Part Two

A PROGRAM TO FOLLOW

V.

Posture

The way you stand, walk, and sit says a very great deal about you. Frequently the first impression you make on others is determined by how you carry yourself.

Poor posture too often contributes to figure problems as well as to health problems. Years of bad posture not only cause rounded shoulders, a protruding tummy, and midriff bulge, but are also responsible for a seeming epidemic of back problems. The common backache annually costs American industry in excess of $1 billion in lost services and goods, plus another $225 million in workmen's compensation. Bad posture puts stress and strain on parts of our anatomy that were not meant to carry the strain; it forces vital organs to assume unnatural positions. A person whose posture is bad cannot hope to look or feel as good as one who practices good posture. The sad thing is that many people have gotten into the habit of bad posture and are not even aware of it. They go through life with a backache and never know why.

With muscles that are kept strong and active it is easier to maintain good posture, to walk tall, and to look your best. The muscle strength, however, is a necessary part of good posture.

Why not take a minute and analyze your posture? Stand as you normally stand. Are your knees straight but relaxed? Are your hips even, not raised or sticking out either side? Is your seat tucked under? Abdomen flat? Torso erect? Neck and head balanced over the body, not thrust forward? Shoulders down? Does your weight feel evenly balanced over your feet? If you can answer yes to all these questions, your posture is close to perfect!

In the past few years I have had the opportunity to work with teenagers, college students, and adults in the area of fitness, figure control, and posture. I have come to believe that many of our posture problems can be solved by a correct head position. In many sports, such as diving, tumbling, acrobatics, and so on, head position is of utmost importance. In these activities it is frequently said that "the body follows the head." I believe this is also true with posture. If the head is erect—as tall as it can be—the rest of the body seems to fall in line; the tummy is in, the hips are tucked in, the chest is high. Try it! Lift the top of your head as if you are trying to touch the ceiling. Do not lift your chin, just the top of your head. Notice the difference? Remind yourself frequently throughout the day to lift the top of your head. It works!

Of course we must have the muscular strength

to hold ourselves erect. These things go together—physical fitness and good posture.

> No good thing will he withhold from them that walk
> uprightly (Psalm 84:11).

VI.

Basic Daily Fitness Program

The next few pages contain what I consider to be a good
basic daily fitness program. It includes an exercise for
each general area of the body, a vigorous activity (no
fitness program is complete without an activity
to build endurance, stamina, and coordination),
and a time of deep breathing and relaxation which
are also a vital part of your time to fitness.

The number of times that you do each exercise and
the rate at which you increase the number of repetitions are included with each exercise explanation.

If you have not exercised in a long time or are
not sure that you are in good health, have a talk
with your doctor before you undertake any program
of physical activity. Chances are he will be delighted
with your decision to improve your health, your
appearance, and your self-image. One eminent
physician was recently quoted as saying that the closest
thing we have at this time to an anti-aging pill is
a good physical fitness program. Take the prescription!

A Program To Follow

The time of day that you exercise is not nearly as important as the regularity with which you do it. Pick a time that is most convenient for you and try to have your fitness time at that same time each day. By exercising at the same time each day it becomes a part of your daily routine—a habit! A mighty good habit!

Basic Daily Fitness Program

39

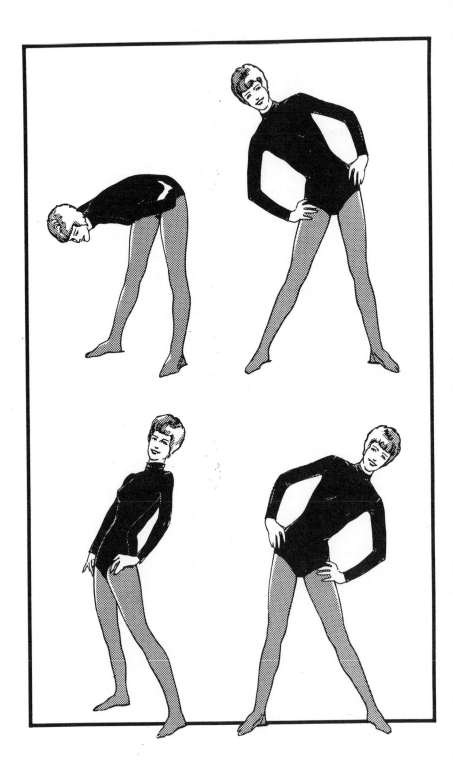

Four Bounces

Stand with your feet approximately shoulder width apart. Hands on hips.

1. Bend forward from the waist and bounce down toward knees for 4 counts.
2. Bend toward right side and bounce directly to side for 4 counts.
3. Bend backward and bounce gently 4 counts.
4. Bend toward left side and bounce 4 counts.

This exercise is a great one to start your day. Its emphasis is on the waistline and midsection, but it is also a good stretch for the back and a tension-reliever.

Start with five sets the first day. After five days begin to add one set each day until you are doing ten sets daily.

This is my commandment, That ye love one another, as I have loved you.

John 15:12

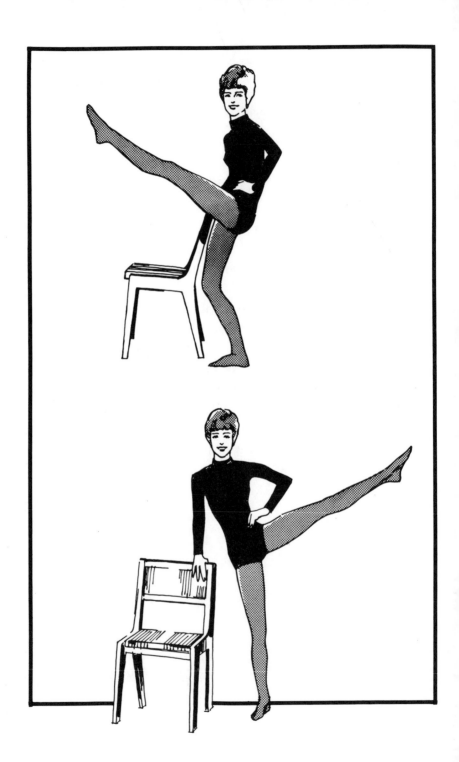

Chair Leg Swings

Stand beside a sturdy straight chair. Lift your leg up and out to the side as far as you can easily. Bring your leg down to starting position; then lift forward and up as far as you can easily, again returning to starting position. Repeat the sequence ten times, to a moderate count of four. Then move to the other side of the chair and repeat with other leg. After five days begin to add one leg swing each day until you are doing twenty leg swings on each side.

An outside thick bulge and a looseness on the inside thigh are common figure problems. This is an exercise to help you solve either or both of these problems.

I will praise thee; for I am fearfully and wonderfully made: marvelous are thy works. . . .

Psalm 139:14

43

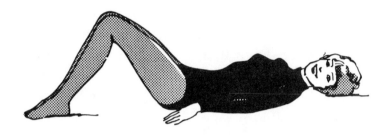

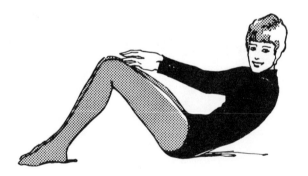

Modified Sit-ups

Lie on the floor on your back with your knees bent, feet flat on the floor.

Curl up, lifting just your head and shoulders, reaching toward your knees with your hands. As you curl up, count slowly to four. Then roll down to a slow count of four.

Do not try to sit all the way up; simply *curl* up, lifting head and shoulders from about the bra line.

This is a very effective exercise for strengthening abdominal muscles. Start with five to ten the first day, then add one each day until you are doing twenty to twenty-five each day. If you are striving for a tighter tummy, this exercise can help!

From the rising of the sun unto the going down of the same the Lord's name is to be praised.

Psalm 113:3

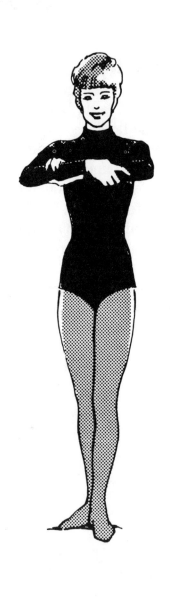

Bust and Arm Push

You may sit or stand as you do this exercise. Just be sure that you practice good posture in either case.

Cross your arms in front of bustline, wrapping fingers around forearms. Push in toward the elbows and hold the contraction for about one second. Release the contraction and repeat. Count each push or contraction as one.

This exercise is very easy to do, yet is very effective. It is perhaps the most often recommended exercise for the bustline. Do 100 pushes each day. It will take very little time (you can do this exercise while you are watching TV, when you are a passenger in a car, or under the hair dryer) and it is time very well spent. It will help to retain or regain upper arm firmness, as well as improve the bustline.

As you do this exercise, concentrate on keeping abdominal muscles tight as an extra help there.

Today if ye will hear his voice.

Psalm 95:7

47

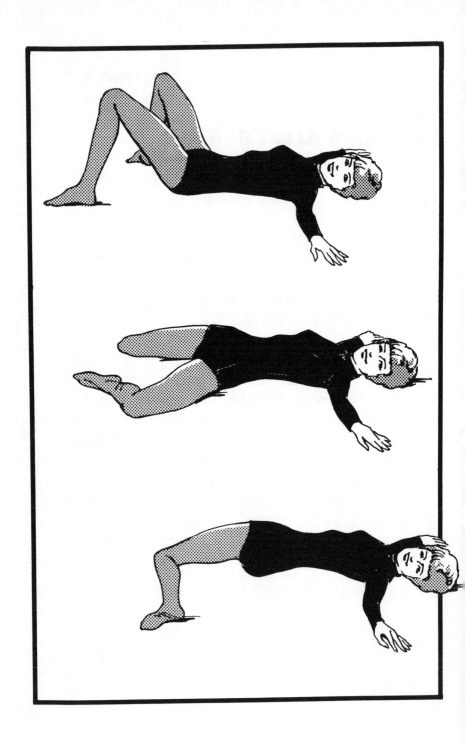

Hip Rolls

Lie on your back on the floor with knees bent and feet flat on the floor. Knees and feet are spread about two feet apart. Keep your arms and shoulders on the floor as you drop both knees to the left side as far as you can easily. Bring your knees back up and over to the right side.

Start with 25 to 50 hip rolls at first and gradually work up to 100 each day, counting the movement each way as one.

The hip area tends to be a problem for many women, especially those whose jobs require a lot of sitting. This exercise is easy to do, but very effective for hips, waist, and abdominal areas.

I also recommend this exercise for men who are beginning to "spread" in the midsection.

This is the day which the Lord hath made; we will rejoice and be glad in it.

Psalm 118:24

49

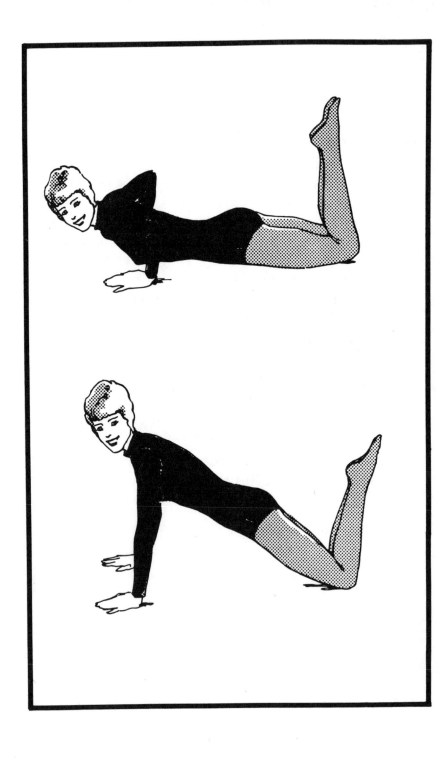

Modified Push-ups

Lie on the floor, face down. Bend your knees so that your toes are pointing toward ceiling. Place your hands on floor under your shoulders with fingers pointing forward. Push your body off the floor until your arms are fully extended. Keep your back straight. Hold for one count and slowly lower to touch your nose lightly to floor. Do not allow your body to touch the floor between push-ups.

Push up and repeat.

You may not have enough upper-arm strength to do more than one or two of these, an indication that you need to build strength there. Start with one to five (as many as you can do at first) and build until you are doing at least ten each day.

This exercise develops muscles that support the breasts, the arms, chest and shoulders.

As the hart panteth after the water brooks, so panteth my soul after thee, O God.

Psalm 42:1

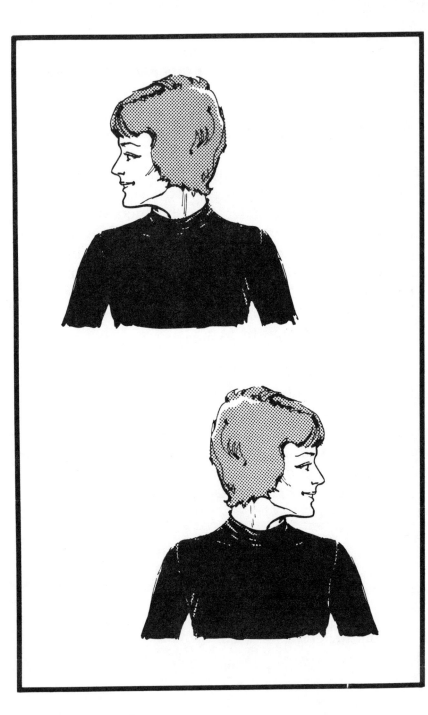

Neck and Eye Exercise

Sit or stand with shoulders very square. Turn your head to the right side as far as you can, as if you were trying to bring your chin over your shoulder. Look as far behind you as possible (pick a spot directly behind you and try to see it from both directions). Turn just the head; do not turn your body.

Repeat movement to left side.

Do this twenty times, counting one each time you turn your head to the side.

Our bodies accumulate tension and we feel it most often in the back of the neck. This exercise will help to release that tension, help firm up the chin and throat, and is also a good exercise for the muscles of the eyes.

I will lift up mine eyes unto the hills, from whence cometh my help.

Psalm 121:1

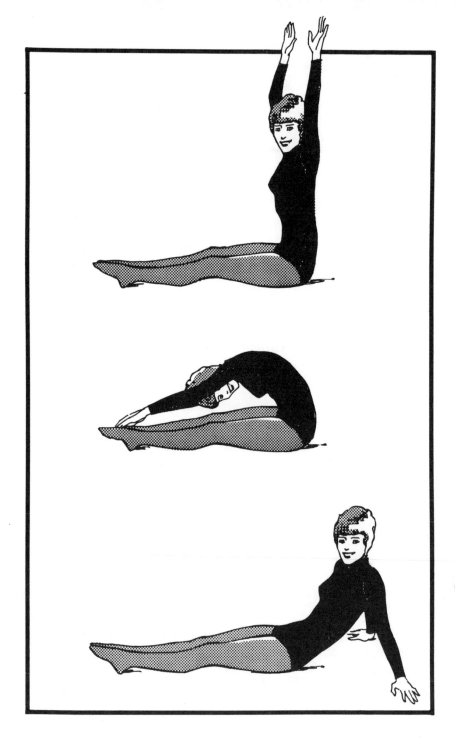

Deep Breathing Stretch

Sit on the floor with legs extended. Reach toward the ceiling with your hands, and, as you do, breathe in deeply. Reach toward toes with your fingers and exhale slowly as you do. Reach up toward ceiling as you inhale slowly. Lean back on hands and exhale slowly.

Repeat several times.

Do not rush this one. It should be a slow, rhythmical movement. Breathe in and out slowly, but do not gulp the air. This exercise is often recommended for expectant mothers. If you are pregnant you *do* need to be exercising. Check with your doctor, find out how much exercise you should be doing and do it!

Because thy lovingkindness is better than life, my lips shall praise thee. Thus will I bless thee while I live: I will lift up my hands in thy name.

Psalm 63:3–4

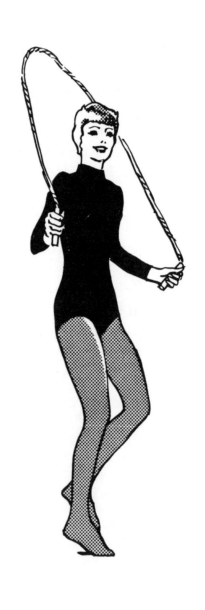

Rope Skipping

A vigorous activity is necessary for a well-rounded fitness program. Skipping rope is a great way to meet that need. Get a good, sturdy, adult-sized skip rope. Be sure that you have the proper length rope for your height. When you stand with both feet on the rope, the handles should come somewhere between just above the waistline and the armpits.

Many fitness authorities are now in agreement that rope skipping is one of the most convenient, least expensive, most effective ways of getting the vigorous exercise that you need each day.

For conditioning purposes it is preferable to skip rope with alternate feet (first one foot forward and then the other). There are many ways to skip rope. You will probably find that you skip with one foot leading forward each time—the way you learned as a child. Chances are you were not taught to skip rope, and you may have to relearn to skip with alternate feet. This may seem a little awkward to you at first, but don't allow that to discourage you. As you skip rope, make the movement rhythmic and relaxed. Skip just high enough to clear the rope and land on the balls of your feet.

I do my daily rope skipping in my kitchen on the

padded kitchen carpet. Any low-pile carpet where you can skip is really ideal. Skipping on a concrete surface is not recommended, but if that is your only possibility be sure to wear well-constructed tennis shoes.

The first day start by skipping just a few times—maybe just 25 repetitions. Add a few each day, working toward 100 skips. After you reach that goal, begin to think in terms of minutes. At a rate of approximately 80 to 100 repetitions a minute, gradually work up to 5 to 10 minutes of continuous rope skipping each day.

Rope skipping is as effective a fitness exercise as you can find—convenient, inexpensive, and fun.

According to my earnest expectation and my hope, that in nothing I shall be ashamed, but that with all boldness, as always, so now also Christ shall be magnified in my body, whether it be by life, or by death.

Philippians 1:20

Relaxation

At the end of your fitness time, plan to spend five minutes of relaxation time.

The importance of this relaxation time cannot be overemphasized. It is an exercise in the release of tensions and self-discipline of the mind and of the body.

Lie on the floor on your back with your arms out to the side, palms up (hands should be approximately twelve to eighteen inches away from the body) in a most comfortable, relaxed position. Allow your feet to fall comfortably apart. Visualize your body position: be sure that your spine is in perfect alignment. Keep this relaxed picture of yourself in your mind throughout your relaxation time.

Practice deep abdominal breathing for the first portion of this time. Breathe through the nostrils with the mouth closed but relaxed. As you inhale, try not to lift the chest; instead, expand the diaphragm and the abdominal area. You might think of the abdomen as a balloon. As you inhale, fill the balloon; as you exhale, totally deflate it. Your exhalation time should be twice as long as inhalation.

It is important to breathe rhythmically. Inhale

59

to a slow count of four, hold for four counts, and then exhale for eight counts.

At the start do only five to six deep breathing rounds. Gradually increase the number until you are spending several minutes ridding your body of the accumulated wastes in your respiratory system. Breathing enthusiast Paul Bragg said: "Oxygen is the greatest of all earthly purifiers."

After you have mastered the technique you can do this "exercise" while walking, standing, sitting, as well as during your relaxation time.

The last portion of the relaxation time is an exercise in mind and body control. You *can* condition your mind and body to relax totally, and, in the doing, rid yourself of much pent-up tension and anxiety. Throughout the deep breathing time you should have retained the original relaxed position *and* the visualization of yourself in that relaxed position.

Starting with your toes, fix your mind on each area of the body and *command* that area to relax. If you are alone, you might even make the command an oral one. Keep your eyes closed and relaxed as you soothingly say to your toes: "Toes, relax, relax, relax. Feet, relax, relax, relax. Calves, relax, relax, relax. Knees. Thighs. Hips. Back. Chest. Shoulders. Arms. Hands. Neck. Face. Scalp." Slowly move from one area to the next, each time focusing your mind completely on that particular area of your body, allowing no other thoughts to enter your mind.

After you have spoken to each area of the body, visualize your total being in that completely relaxed state. Picture the most tranquil place that your mind can imagine and in your mind go there. As you visualize your "perfect spot," be very specific about every detail. May I describe my spot to you? It is early summer on the side of a lush green mountain. The slope is very gentle in "my place." There is a brook that makes a soothing, babbling sound as it moves across its bed of beautiful, smooth stones. Wild daisies are blooming everywhere; big yellow butterflies flit from flower to flower; the sky is radiantly blue and filled with billowy snow-white clouds. In the distance I can hear the ocean as the waves break on the rocks below. I am suspended just above the grass beside the brook. I can smell the grass and feel its coolness reaching toward me. The sun's rays warm my body and there is a soft summer breeze drifting over me. I am filled with the peace that fills this place where I "go" to relax.

If you like my place you are welcome to it, but chances are you will want to change it to your specifications. Once you have found your own place, you can go there instantly to relax and rejuvenate.

You must learn to dwell on even the minute details of your visualization. Do not allow your mind to wander. This will be the most difficult part in the beginning, because most of us have not learned to channel and control our thoughts. We allow them to flit around aimlessly—much as our big yellow butterflies do—from one thing to another. If you find yourself thinking about something other than your relaxed body in your garden of tranquility, immediately pull your thoughts back. After a bit of practice *you* will have control.

The Scriptures tell us that the way to real peace is through total submission to Christ. Paul reminds us to fill our minds with beautiful, good thoughts:

> Always be full of joy in the Lord; I say it again, rejoice! Let everyone see that you are unselfish and considerate in all you do. Remember that the Lord is coming soon. Don't worry about anything; instead, pray about everything; tell God your needs and don't forget to thank him for his answers. If you do this you will experience God's peace, which is far more wonderful than the human mind can understand. His peace will keep your thoughts and your hearts quiet and at rest as you trust in Christ Jesus.
>
> . . . Fix your thoughts on what is true and good and right. Think about things that are pure and lovely, and dwell on the fine, good things in others. Think about all you can praise God for and be glad about . . . and the God of peace will be with you" (Phil. 4:4–9, *Living Bible*) .

VII.

Additional Exercises for Special Figure Problems

After you have been doing the Basic Daily Fitness
   Program for two to three weeks, you may wish
   to begin to add extra exercises for those special
   figure problem areas. The following exercises are
   excellent ones to help you solve some of those figure
   problems.

   Continue to do the basic program in the
   sequence that you have been doing them and add
   the extras just before you skip rope.

   You might also consider doing the extras at another
   time during the day—perhaps while you are watching
   television in the evening. You could easily do an
   extra one hundred hip rolls and thirty or so back
   leg lifts if you are trying to firm up the hip area,
   for instance.

   Exercises and areas concentrated on in this section
   are listed on page 65.

Additional Exercises for Special Figure Problems

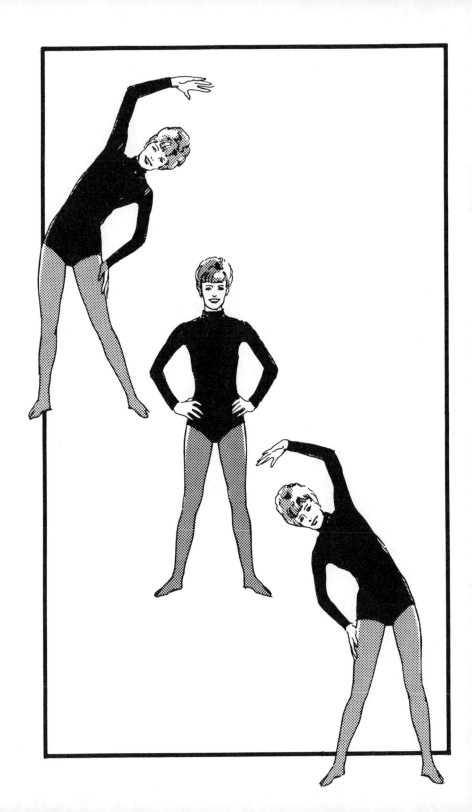

Waist Stretch

Stand with your feet apart, one hand on hip, the other hand over head with palm toward head. Bend directly to side as far as you can stretch easily . . . then give an extra stretch.

Repeat to other side.

This is fun when done to music. Any record with a good beat will do. Spend about two to three minutes each day doing the waist stretch and watch the midriff bulge go. This exercise will also help to release some of those accumulated tensions.

Now glory be to God who by his mighty power at work within us is able to do far more than we would ever dare to ask or even dream of—infinitely beyond our highest prayers, desires, thoughts, or hopes.

Ephesians 3:20 (Living Bible)

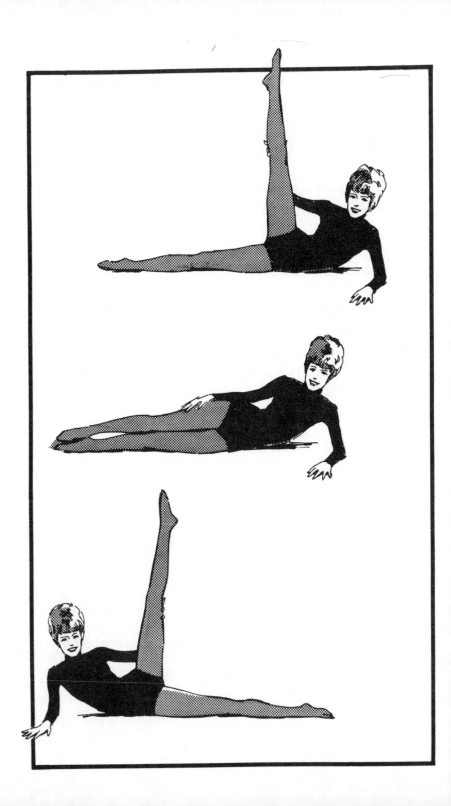

Side Leg Lift

Lie on the floor on your side. Lift your top leg directly up to the side to a slow count of four. Bring the leg down again to a slow count of four. This should be a slow, controlled movement. Lift as far as you can easily, and don't be discouraged if that isn't very far at first. As you increase strength and flexibility you will be able to lift further. Start with ten leg lifts on each side and gradually work up to twenty to thirty on each side.

This exercise tightens inside and outside thigh areas. If you have looseness or a bulge in the thigh area, this is a good exercise to add to your daily exercise program.

Create in me a clean heart, O God; and renew a right spirit within me.

Psalm 51:10

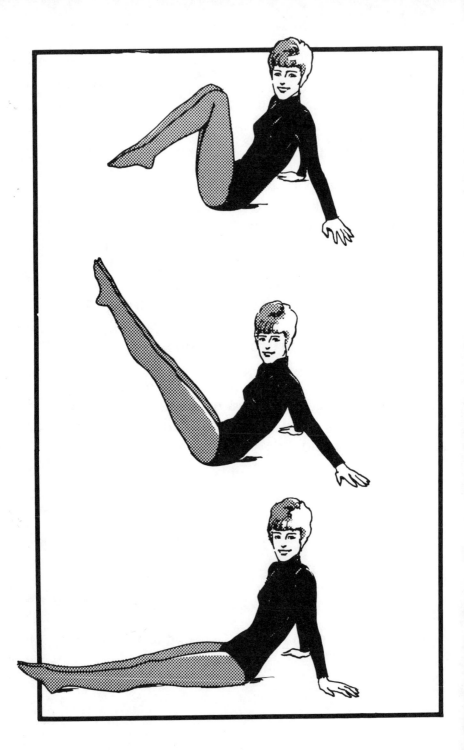

Sitting–Knees to Chest

Sit on the floor. Lean back on your hands and bring your knees close to your chest. Extend your legs up and out with toes pointed. Slowly lower legs until they rest on the floor. Bring knees back to chest and repeat.

Start with five of these; add one each day until you are doing twenty to twenty-five each day.

If you are serious about tightening abdominal muscles, this is a good extra exercise for you to add to your daily exercise program.

Also be sure that you are practicing good posture. Poor posture often contributes to a protruding tummy.

Rejoice in the Lord alway: and again I say, rejoice.
Philippians 4:4

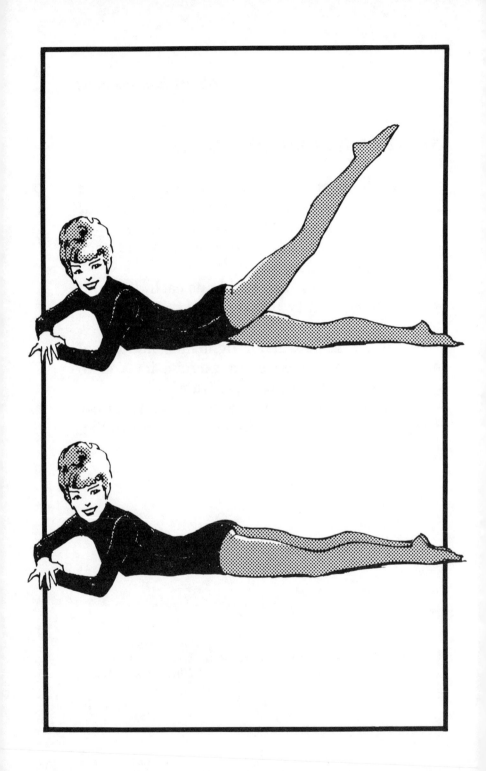

Back Leg Lift

Lie on the floor face down. You may either rest your head on your hands or lift it. Slowly lift your right leg directly up in the back as far as you can easily, keeping the leg straight. Bring right leg down and repeat with left leg.

Start with twenty lifts, alternating legs. Do this several days and then begin to add two lifts each day until you are doing forty to fifty each day.

This exercise will help to tighten and trim both the hip and abdominal areas. It also helps to strengthen and release tensions from the lower back.

Arise, shine; for thy light is come, and the glory of the Lord is risen upon thee.

Isaiah 60:1

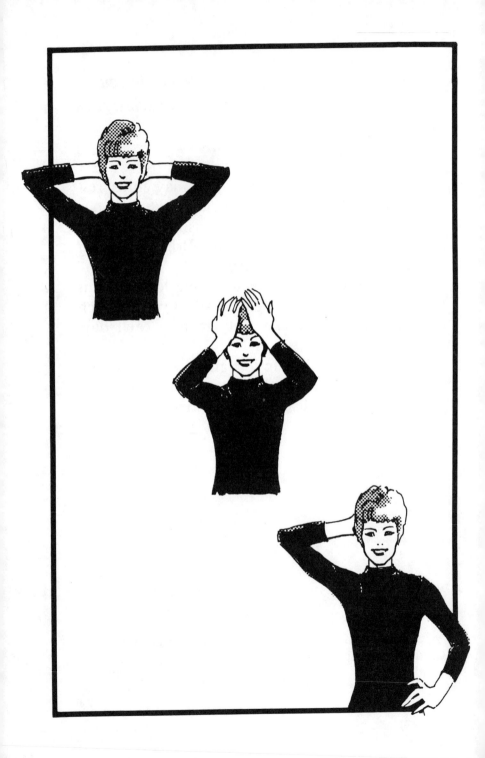

Resistive Neck

Sit or stand with fingers laced behind the head. Pull hands forward and resist the force with the head. Slowly count to six as you hold the contraction; then relax.

Place heels of hands on forehead. Push with hands, resist with head. Hold for six counts. Place palm of left hand on side of head. Push with hand; resist with head. Hold for six counts. Repeat on right side.

Start with four sets and work up to six gradually.

An area that is too often neglected is the neck, chin, and throat. This exercise will help to firm these areas as well as relieve tension in the back of the neck, *and* you get a bonus in strengthened upper arms.

Let the field be joyful, and all that is therein; then shall all the trees of the wood rejoice.

Psalm 96:12

75

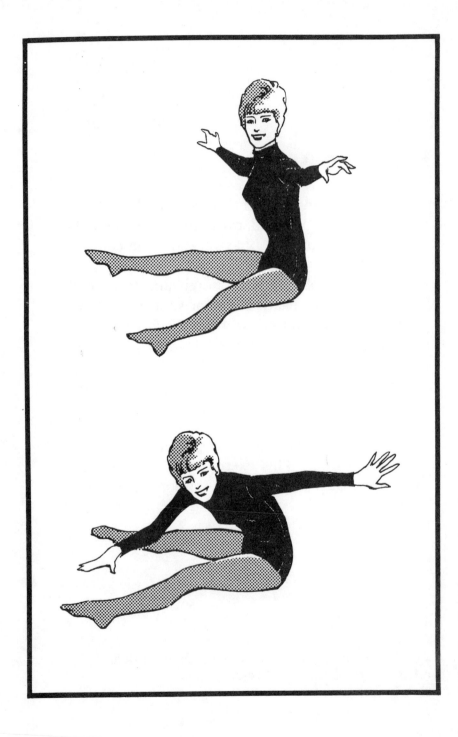

Windmill

Sit with your legs spread far apart, your back tall, and arms reaching out to the sides. Twist your body to the side and try to touch your right foot with your left hand. Return to starting position and repeat action to other side.

The Windmill is a good stretching exercise. It helps to keep an active, trim waistline and mid-section, and it is also good for back flexibility. As you do this exercise be sure that you "sit tall" between movements. Start with twenty of these and gradually work up to fifty.

But thou, O Lord, art a shield for me; my glory, and the lifter up of mine head.

Psalm 3:3

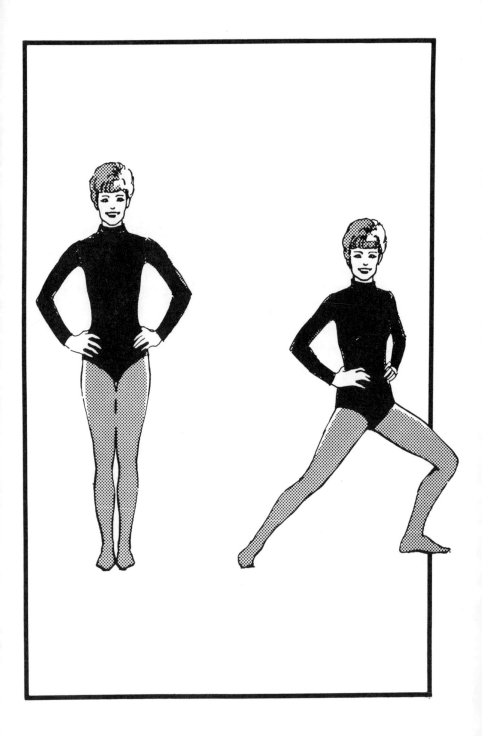

Lunge

Stand with feet side by side. Turn right foot to side and lunge to the side. Bounce in lunge position twice. Return to starting position and lunge to left side. Bounce twice.

Start with five lunges on each side. Add one each day until you are doing fifteen to twenty on each side.

Do not do too many of these at first. This is a "sneaky" exercise and will make you sore if you overdo. It is very effective for that inside thigh looseness and outside thigh bulge. If you are serious about improving your legs, this exercise can help.

The earth is the Lord's and the fulness thereof; the world, and they that dwell therein.

Psalm 24:1

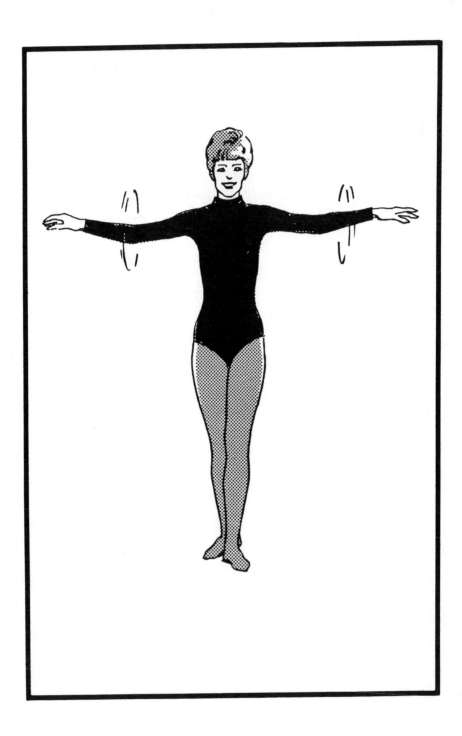

Little Arm Circles

Stand very tall with your arms held out at shoulder level, palms down, feet comfortably apart. Make small circles with your arms. Count eight circles in one direction and eight back the other way.

Turn your palms up and repeat the circles, eight times each direction.

Repeat the entire exercise four times at a rather rapid tempo.

The upper arm area requires special attention. Since we don't do the kind of activities in our daily routines that would keep these muscles active, we must make that activity with a planned exercise time. This exercise helps.

As you do this exercise, think about your posture. Stand as tall as you know you should. Practice good posture at all times!

Lead me in thy truth, and teach me: for thou art the God of my salvation; on thee do I wait all the day.
Psalm 25:5

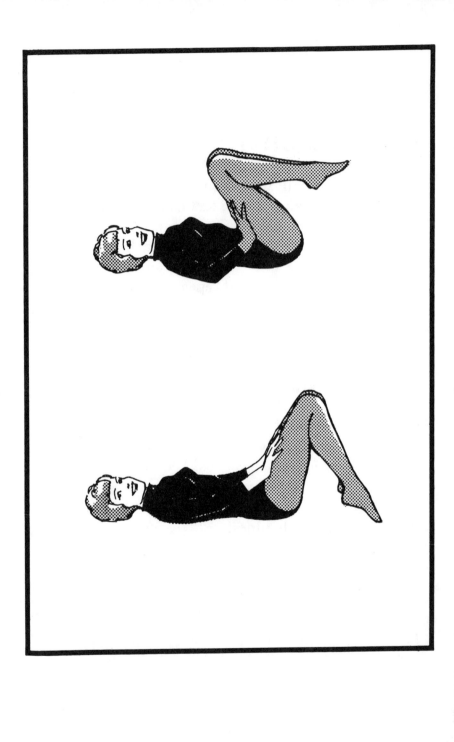

Resistive Tummy

This is an isometric exercise for the abdominal area. An isometric exercise is one in which you resist a force—in this case, your own force. Lie on your back with your knees drawn up toward your chest. Place your hands on your thighs.

1. Push against your legs with your hands and resist the push with the legs. To the slow count of six push legs down until toes touch the floor.
2. Release contraction.
3. Bring knees up again, resisting your own force all the way, to a slow count of six.
4. Release contraction.

Repeat ten times.

You determine how easy or how difficult this exercise is by how hard you push against yourself. At first you should make it easy. Push hard enough that you feel the muscles working, but don't make it difficult. As you continue to exercise each day, you gradually increase the amount of force you use until you are working quite hard.

This is a great exercise to start with if you've had a baby recently or abdominal surgery and need something easy to help you begin to regain abdominal strength and tone.

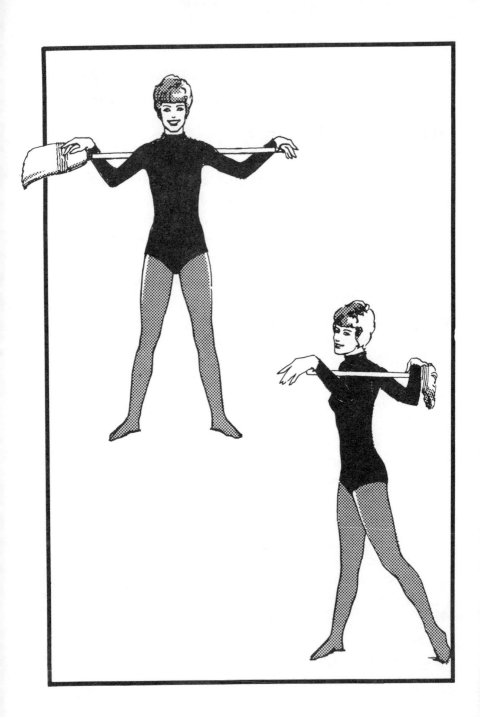

Broom Twist

Stand with your feet spread apart. Place broom just behind your shoulders and hang your hands over the broom handle (pretend you're a scarecrow).

Twist to the right side as far as you can easily and then give a little extra push; swing and push.

Repeat movement to the left side.

A good twisting, stretching exercise. If your posture is not as good as it should be, make this an exercise that you do each day. It is very effective and *feels* so good. Start with ten to twenty swings and gradually work up to forty or fifty.

The broom twist exercise is especially good for the muscles in the back and shoulders, and also the waistline and midsection.

Show me thy ways, O Lord; teach me thy paths.
Psalm 25:4

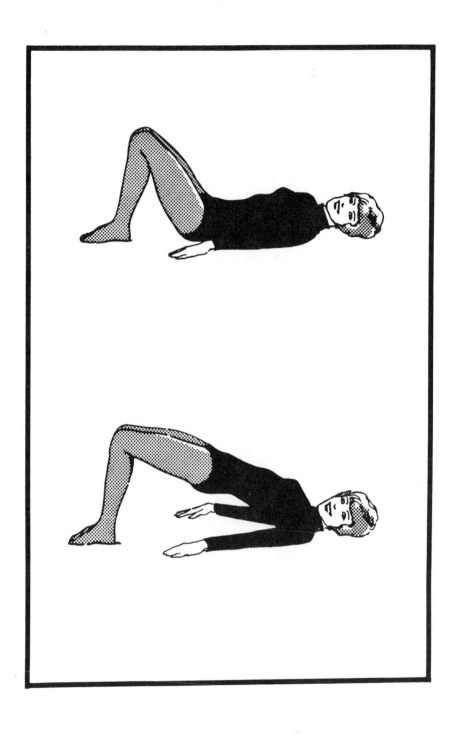

Hip Raises

Lie on your back with arms beside your body; palms down, knees bent, and feet flat on the floor. Slowly lift your hips until your body is in a straight line from knees to shoulders. Hold the position for a slow count of five. Slowly lower the back from the top down as if you are lowering one vertebra at a time.

Repeat five to ten times.

I would urge every woman to do this exercise every day. It helps strengthen back, abdominal muscles, and hips. Why not do this one during the commercial breaks of your favorite television program *instead* of going for snacks?

O magnify the Lord with me, and let us exalt his name together.

Psalm 34:3

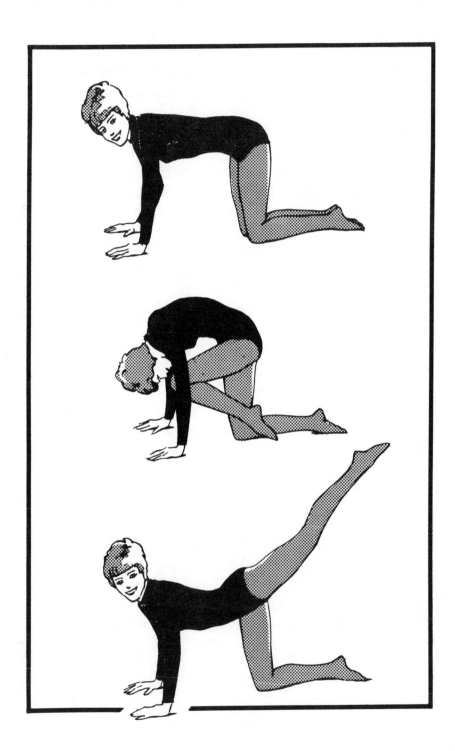

Old Gray Mare

Start on your hands and knees on the floor. Bring one knee up under the chest and then try to touch your nose to your knee. Kick the leg up and out in the back as you lift up your head.

Repeat six times with each leg.

This exercise is called the "Old Gray Mare," and it is a good one. It is good for the hips, the legs, and the *plus* includes back, chin and throat.

Know ye that the Lord he is God: it is he that hath made us, and not we ourselves; we are his people, and the sheep of his pasture.

Psalm 100:3

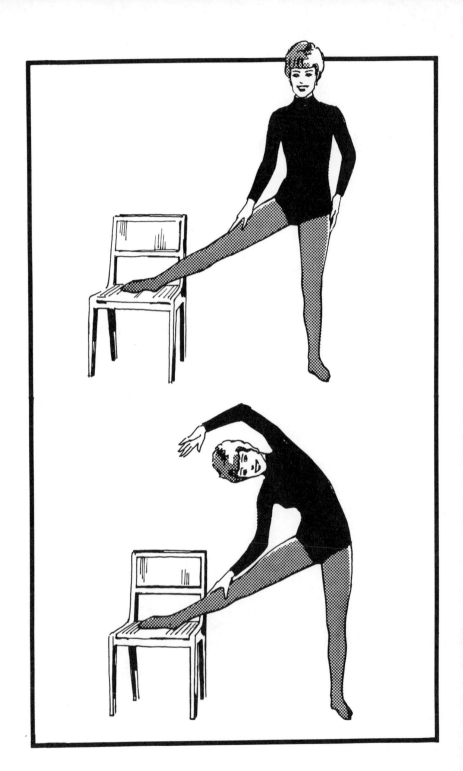

Chair Waist Stretch

Stand beside a good sturdy chair. Place one foot securely in the chair. Bring the arm that is outside up over your head as you bend directly to the side, getting a long stretch all the way down the side. You will feel a delightful stretch in the inside thigh area also. Return to starting position and repeat ten times.

Move to other side of chair and repeat on other side.

In order to look and feel your best you *must* get a certain amount of exercise every day. Set aside a few minutes each day. Do an exercise for each area of the body. Make your daily exercise time a habit. You'll look better, feel better, and like yourself better.

Seek ye first the kingdom of God, and his righteousness. . . .

Matthew 6:33

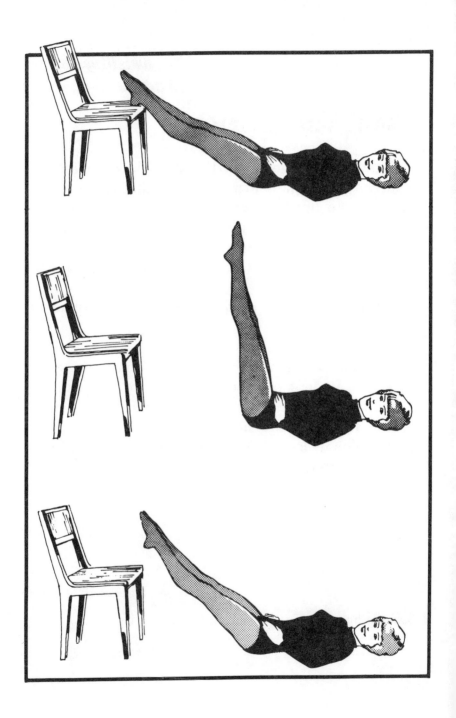

Feet in Chair

Lie on the floor with heels resting on the seat of a straight chair. Lift legs, reaching toward the ceiling with your toes. Slowly lower legs to rest in chair.

If your goal is a flatter tummy, here is help. Do this exercise five times today. Add one each day until you are doing fifteen to twenty each day. Regular exercise is your key to a healthier, happier, more attractive you!

Therefore the redeemed of the Lord shall return,
and come with singing unto Zion; and everlasting joy
shall be upon their head: they shall obtain gladness and
joy; and sorrow and mourning shall flee away.
Isaiah 51:11

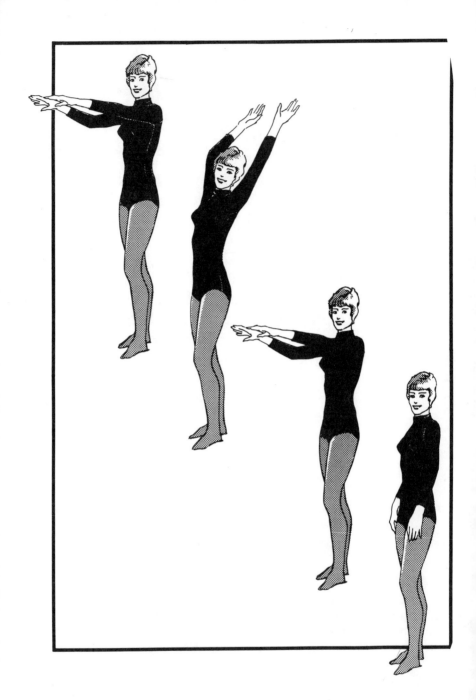

Arm Exercise

Stand tall with your arms by your sides. On the count of one, lift arms to shoulder level in front of your body. On the count of two lift arms as far up and back as you can easily. You should feel a good, long stretch. On three, bring arms back to shoulder level. On four, back to starting position.

Repeat ten times.

A great waker-upper, this exercise is very good for the arms, shoulders, back, and entire torso area. It might be a good one with which to start your fitness time, helping to get some of the "kinks" out and start moving.

And Jesus said unto him, No man, having put his hand to the plough, and looking back, is fit for the kingdom of God.

Luke 9:62